# Protein Shakes

## Top 50 Protein Shake Recipes for Weight Loss

### By
### Bring On Fitness

*Bring On Fitness*

© **Copyright 2018 – Bring On Fitness – All rights reserved.**

The contents of this book may not be reproduced, duplicated, or transmitted without direct written permission from the author.

Under no circumstances will any legal responsibility or blame be held against the publisher for any reparation, damages, or monetary loss due to the information herein, either directly or indirectly.

**Legal Notice:**

This book is copyright protected. This is only for personal use. You cannot amend, distribute, sell, use, quote, or paraphrase any part or the content of this book without the consent of the author.

**Disclaimer Notice:**

Please note the information contained in this document is for educational and entertainment purposes only. Every attempt has been made to provide accurate, up-to-date, complete, and reliable information. No warranties of any kind are expressed or implied. Readers acknowledge that the author is not engaging in the rendering of legal, financial, medical, or professional advice. The content of this book has been derived from various sources. Please consult a licensed professional before attempting any techniques outlined in this book.

By reading this document, the reader agrees that under no circumstances is the author responsible for any losses, direct or indirect, which are incurred as a result of the use of information contained within this document, including, but not limited to, errors, omissions, or inaccuracies.

*Bring On Fitness*

## About Bring On Fitness

Our passion for fitness gave life to **Bring On Fitness**. We started with the goal of helping as many people as we can. To educate, motivate and to help change peoples lives for the better. Bring On Fitness is not only for the fitness enthusiasts, but also for the beginner. We strongly believe nothing is more important than learning the basics and creating a strong foundation in both nutrition - through meal planning, and in exercise - by following a specific plan. This is just as important for the beginner, as it is for the experienced athlete.

We set high standards for ourselves, the information we share, and the products we carry. Our goal is to provide you with exceptional products that suit your needs and the knowledge and motivation to help you work towards and achieve your health and fitness goals.

Check us out at www.bringonfitness.com

*"Our Mission is to have a positive impact in changing peoples lives. We will deliver the best possible fitness and nutrition solutions that will empower people to achieve their health and fitness goals."*

*Bring On Fitness*

# Table of Contents

**Introduction** ......................................................................... 11

**Chapter One: Fruit Based Shakes** ........................... 13

    Vanilla Yogurt and Blueberry Smoothie .............................. 13

    Strawberry Banana Shake ....................................................... 14

    Blueberry Tofu High Protein Smoothie ............................... 15

    Sunrise Smoothie ..................................................................... 16

    Banana, Orange and Carrot Shake ........................................ 17

    Spinach Flax Protein Smoothie ............................................. 18

    Mango Pineapple and Banana Smoothie ............................ 19

    Decadent Vanilla Almond Protein Smoothie ..................... 20

    Super food Shake ..................................................................... 21

    Mango Lassi ............................................................................... 22

    Strawberry Banana Post-Workout Shake ........................... 23

    Tropical Power Shake .............................................................. 24

    Raspberry Banana Chia Smoothie ........................................ 25

    Cherry Ginger Lime Smoothie .............................................. 26

    Apple-Kale Green Smoothie .................................................. 27

**Chapter Two: Chocolate and Coffee Based Shakes** .. 29

    Chocolate Cherry Shake ......................................................... 29

*Bring On Fitness*

    Double Chocolate Mint Smoothie ............................... 30

    Vietnamese Coffee Protein Shake.................................31

    Coffee Lovers Protein Shake......................................... 32

    Mocha Protein Shake..................................................... 33

    Chocolate Raspberry Chia Shake................................. 34

    Chocolate Peanut Butter Smoothie ............................. 35

**Chapter Three: Breakfast Shakes .......................... 37**

    Greek Goddess Banana Oat Protein Shake ....................... 37

    French Toast Shake .......................................................38

    Blueberry Breakfast Shake ........................................... 39

    Chocolate Peanut Butter Banana Breakfast Shake ............. 40

    Apple and Great Gains Shake........................................ 41

    Chia Seed Piña Colada ................................................. 42

**Chapter Four: Dessert Shakes ................................ 43**

    Key Lime Pie Protein Shake ......................................... 43

    Vanilla Pumpkin Pie Shake .......................................... 45

    Black Forest Protein Shake........................................... 46

    High Protein Oreo Milkshake....................................... 47

    Orange Julius.................................................................48

    Oatmeal Raisin "Cookie" in a Glass............................. 49

    Orange Creamsicle........................................................50

## Chapter Five: Nut Based Shakes .......................... 51

Peanut Butter – Banana Shake ............................................. 51

Very Berry Super Shake ....................................................... 52

Peachy Keen Smoothie ........................................................ 53

Peanut Butter and Jelly Protein Smoothie ........................ 54

Chocolate, Peanut Butter and Banana .............................. 55

Apple Shake ........................................................................... 56

Coconut and Almond Shake ............................................... 57

Almond Butter Chia Shake ................................................. 58

## Chapter Six: Vegan Shakes ...................................... 59

Peanut Butter Cup ................................................................ 59

## Vanilla Chai ............................................................... 60

Dark Chocolate Peppermint Protein Shake ..................... 61

Green Monster ...................................................................... 62

Matcha Pear Green Protein Shake .................................... 63

Baked Apple Shake .............................................................. 64

Toasted Coconut Protein Shake ........................................ 65

## Conclusion .............................................................. 67

*Bring On Fitness*

# Introduction

I want to thank you for choosing this book, *'Protein Shakes: Top 50 Protein Shake Recipes for Weight Loss.'* I hope you will find the recipes delicious and that they are helpful in your weight loss journey.

Losing weight and becoming fit are two of the major goals that many people aspire to achieve. We all want a great looking, fit and healthy body, and must be willing to work hard for it. It is impossible to sculpt a great body without hard work, in both your diet and working out routine.

Working out is not always easy, making time to spend 60 minutes in the gym can be challenge; not to mention the time it takes to prepare your meals on a daily basis.

Dieting can be difficult, as you may need to cut out your favorite foods, and some diets even require you to significantly cut down on food, leaving you hungry most of the time. Not many of us are ready to let go of delicious tasting foods. So it is no wonder why people fail in the first few weeks of a new diet.

There are many diets to try and most will require you to cut out certain foods from your meals. But what if I told you that you can diet without compromising all the taste?

In this book, you can find a variety of recipes for protein shakes and smoothies that are not only delicious but are extremely healthy. These smoothies are rich, tasty and refreshing. They will keep you full for a long time and you won't feel hungry for hours, which will help you avoid empty calories and allow you to better stick to your diet.

*Bring On Fitness*

So what are you waiting for? Follow the recipes in this book and experience weight loss in the healthiest manner, without starving your body.

Thanks again for purchasing this book. I hope you enjoy it!

# Chapter One: Fruit Based Shakes

## Vanilla Yogurt and Blueberry Smoothie

Serves: 2

### Nutritional values per serving:

- Calories – 443
- Fat – 14.5 g
- Carbohydrate – 63 g
- Protein – 18 g

### Ingredients:

- 2 cups fresh blueberries
- 2 cups skim milk or soy milk
- 2 tablespoons flaxseed oil
- 12 ounces vanilla yogurt
- Ice cubes, as required

### Method:

1. Add all the ingredients except flaxseed oil into a blender and blend for 30-40 seconds or until smooth
2. Pour into tall glasses. Add flaxseed oil, stir and serve right away.

*Bring On Fitness*

# Strawberry Banana Shake

Serves: 2

## Nutritional values per serving:

- Calories – 409
- Fat – 9 g
- Carbohydrate – 47 g
- Protein – 55 g

## Ingredients:

- 1 ½ cups water
- 2 cups frozen strawberries
- 2 cups spinach
- 2 bananas, peeled, sliced, frozen
- 4 tablespoons ground flaxseeds
- 4 scoops vanilla protein powder

## Method:

1. Add water, berries, spinach, yogurt, flaxseeds, walnuts and protein powder into a blender and blend for 30-40 seconds or until smooth.
2. Pour into tall glasses and serve with crushed ice.

# Blueberry Tofu High Protein Smoothie

Serves: 2

## Nutritional values per serving: 18 ounces

- Calories – 425
- Fat – 11 g
- Carbohydrate – 83 g
- Protein – 21 g

## Ingredients:

- 1 1/3 cups blueberries
- 2 cups soy milk
- 2 tablespoons honey
- 2 medium bananas
- 12 ounces soft silken tofu

## Method:

1. Add blueberries, soymilk, honey, bananas and tofu into the blender.
2. Blend for 30-40 seconds or until smooth.
3. Pour into tall glasses and serve with crushed ice.

## Sunrise Smoothie

Serves: 2

### Nutritional values per serving:

- Calories – 209
- Fats – 1.8 g
- Carbohydrate – 42 g
- Protein – 8 g

### Ingredients:

- 2 bananas, sliced, frozen
- 2 cups frozen mixed berries
- 2 oranges, peeled, separated into segments, deseeded
- 10 ounces vanilla Greek yogurt

### Method:

1. Add all the ingredients into a blender.
2. Blend for 30-40 seconds or until smooth.
3. Pour into a tall glass and serve with crushed ice.

# Banana, Orange and Carrot Shake

Serves: 2

**Nutritional values per serving:**

- Calories – 378
- Fat – 12 g
- Carbohydrate – 58 g
- Protein – 17 g

**Ingredients:**

- 2 bananas, peeled, sliced
- 1 orange, peeled, separated into segments, deseeded
- 3 cups spinach, torn
- 2 carrots, chopped
- 1 teaspoon pumpkin seeds
- 1 teaspoon hemp seeds
- 2 teaspoons ground flaxseeds
- 1 cup Greek yogurt
- 1 cup low fat milk

**Method:**

1. Add all the ingredients into a blender.
2. Blend for 30-40 seconds or until smooth.
3. Pour into a tall glass and serve with crushed ice.

*Bring On Fitness*

## Spinach Flax Protein Smoothie

Serves: 2

### Nutritional values per serving:

- Calories – 231
- Fat – 8 g
- Carbohydrates – 23 g
- Protein – 19 g

### Ingredients:

- 2 cups almond milk, unsweetened
- ½ cup frozen pineapple
- ½ cup frozen mango chunks
- 1 banana, peeled, sliced
- 2 tablespoons chia seeds
- 2 tablespoons flax meal (optional)
- 2 cups baby spinach
- 2 scoops vanilla protein powder

### Method:

1. Add milk, the fruit, chia seeds, flax meal, spinach and protein powder into a blender.
2. Blend for 30-40 seconds or until smooth.
3. Pour into glasses and serve.
4. Serve with crushed ice.

# Mango Pineapple and Banana Smoothie

Serves: 2

**Nutritional values per serving:**

- Calories – 198.6
- Fat – 1.3 g
- Carbohydrate – 31.4 g
- Protein – 20.5 g

**Ingredients:**

- ½ cup frozen mango pieces
- ½ cup frozen pineapple pieces
- 1 small banana, peeled, sliced
- 1 cup skim milk
- ½ cup fat free yogurt
- 1 scoop vanilla whey protein powder
- Sweetener of your choice (optional)

**Method:**

1. Add all the ingredients into a blender.
2. Blend for about 30-40 seconds or until smooth.
3. Pour into tall glasses and serve with crushed ice.

*Bring On Fitness*

# Decadent Vanilla Almond Protein Smoothie

Serves: 2

## Nutritional values per serving:

- Calories – 255
- Fat – 10 g
- Carbohydrate – 28 g
- Protein – 22 g

## Ingredients:

- 2 scoops vanilla protein powder
- ½ cup fat free vanilla yogurt
- 1 ½ cups vanilla almond milk, unsweetened
- 1 banana, peeled, sliced, frozen
- 2 tablespoons nut butter of your choice
- Ice cubes, as required

<u>Toppings:</u> Use any

- Almonds, slivered
- Ground cinnamon
- Flaxseeds

## Method:

1. Add protein powder, yogurt, milk, banana, nut butter and ice into a blender.
2. Blend for about 30-40 seconds or until smooth.
3. Pour into tall glasses.
4. Sprinkle toppings sand serve with crushed ice.

## Super food Shake

Serves: 2

### Nutritional values per serving:

- Calories – 329
- Fat – 4 g
- Carbohydrate – 52 g
- Protein – 28 g

### Ingredients:

- 1 cup frozen cherries, pitted
- 1 cup frozen strawberries
- 1 cup beets, peeled, chopped
- 1 banana, peeled, sliced
- 2 tablespoons ground flaxseeds
- 2 cups water
- 2 scoops chocolate whey protein powder
- Ice cubes, as required

### Method:

1. Add protein powder, water, cherries, strawberries, beets, banana, flaxseeds, and ice into a blender.
2. Blend for about 30-40 seconds or until smooth.
3. Pour into tall glasses and serve.

## Mango Lassi

Serves: 2

**Nutritional values per serving:**

- Calories – 200
- Fat – 1.5 g
- Carbohydrate – 26 g
- Protein – 18 g

**Ingredients:**

- 1 ½ cups mango pieces (fresh or frozen)
- 1 cup cold water
- 1 teaspoon maple syrup
- ¼ teaspoon ground cardamom
- 1 ½ cups nonfat Greek yogurt
- 1 cup lemon juice
- 2 teaspoons chopped pistachio
- ¼ teaspoon vanilla extract

**Method:**

1. Add mango, water, maple syrup, cardamom, yogurt, lemon juice and vanilla into a blender.
2. Blend for about 30-40 seconds or until smooth.
3. Pour into tall glasses.
4. Sprinkle pistachio on top sand serve with crushed ice.

# Strawberry Banana Post-Workout Shake

Serves: 2

## Nutritional values per serving:

- Calories – 489
- Fat – 11 g
- Carbohydrate – 59 g
- Protein – 39 g

## Ingredients:

- 2 cups strawberries, chopped
- 2 cups plain low fat kefir
- 2 bananas, peeled, sliced
- ¼ cup walnuts, chopped
- 2 scoops vanilla whey protein powder

## Method:

1. Add all the ingredients into a blender.
2. Blend for about 30-40 seconds or until smooth.
3. Pour into tall glasses and serve with crushed ice.

## Tropical Power Shake

Serves: 2

**Nutritional values per serving: With water**

- Calories – 525
- Fat – 12 g
- Carbohydrate – 46 g
- Protein – 58 g

**Ingredients:**

- 3 cups water or milk
- 1 banana, peeled, sliced
- 2 cups spinach
- 2 cups pineapple chunks
- ¼ cup coconut flakes, unsweetened
- 4 scoops vanilla protein powder
- 2 tablespoons ground flaxseeds
- 1 cup plain yogurt

**Method:**

1. Add all the ingredients into a blender.
2. Blend for about 30-40 seconds or until smooth.
3. Pour into tall glasses and serve with crushed ice.

## Raspberry Banana Chia Smoothie

Serves: 2

**Nutritional values per serving:**

- Calories – 268
- Fat – 5.6 g
- Carbohydrate – 34.1 g
- Protein – 24.3 g

**Ingredients:**

- 1 cup raspberries
- 1 banana, peeled, sliced
- 1 cup plain Greek yogurt
- 2 scoops protein powder
- 2 tablespoons chia seeds
- 1 teaspoon ground cinnamon
- 2 cups ice
- 1 cup water
- 1/8 teaspoon ground nutmeg

**Method:**

1. Add all the ingredients into a blender.
2. Blend for about 30-40 seconds or until smooth.
3. Pour into tall glasses and serve with crushed ice.

*Bring On Fitness*

# Cherry Ginger Lime Smoothie

Serves: 2

**Nutritional values per serving:**

- Calories – 320
- Fat – 2.8 g
- Carbohydrate – 58.8 g
- Protein – 7.8 g

**Ingredients:**

- 1 cup cherries, fresh or frozen, pitted
- 1 tablespoon tart cherry juice
- ½ lime, peeled
- ½ cup blueberries, fresh or frozen
- 1/3 cup plain Greek yogurt
- ¼ green apple, cored
- 1 inch fresh ginger root, peeled, thinly sliced
- 1 tablespoon flaxseeds
- Ice cubes, as required
- 1 scoop protein powder
- ½ cup water

**Method:**

1. Add all the ingredients into a blender.
2. Blend for about 30-40 seconds or until smooth.
3. Pour into tall glasses and serve with crushed ice.

*Protein Shakes*

# Apple-Kale Green Smoothie

Serves: 2

## Nutritional values per serving:

- Calories – 291
- Fat – 6 g
- Carbohydrate – 34 g
- Protein – 28 g

## Ingredients:

- 2 cups almond milk, unsweetened
- 2 mini cucumbers, chopped
- 1 large green apple, cored, chopped
- 2 cups almond milk, unsweetened
- 2 scoops vanilla protein powder
- 2 teaspoons lemon juice

## Method:

1. Add all the ingredients into a blender.
2. Blend for about 30-40 seconds or until smooth.
3. Pour into tall glasses and serve with crushed ice.

*Bring On Fitness*

# Chapter Two: Chocolate and Coffee Based Shakes

## Chocolate Cherry Shake

Serves: 2

**Nutritional values per serving:**

- Calories – 500
- Fat – 13 g
- Carbohydrate – 47 g
- Protein – 56 g

**Ingredients:**

- 1 ½ cups water
- 4 cups sweet, dark cherries, pitted
- 2 tablespoons walnuts
- 2 tablespoons cacao nibs or dark cocoa powder
- 4 scoops chocolate protein powder
- 2 cups spinach
- 2 tablespoons ground flaxseeds

**Method:**

1. Add all the ingredients into a blender.
2. Blend for 30-40 seconds or until smooth.
3. Pour into tall glasses and serve with crushed ice.

*Bring On Fitness*

# Double Chocolate Mint Smoothie

Serves: 2

## Nutritional values per serving:

- Calories – 292
- Fat – 12 g
- Carbohydrate – 32 g
- Protein – 25 g

## Ingredients:

- ½ cup water
- 2 tablespoons walnuts
- 2 tablespoons cacao nibs
- 4 tablespoons cocoa powder, unsweetened
- 4 scoops chocolate protein powder
- 1 ½ cups dark chocolate almond milk
- A handful mint leaves
- Ice cubes, as required

## Method:

1. Add water, walnuts, cacao nibs, cocoa, protein powder, almond milk, mint leaves and ice into a blender.
2. Blend for 30-40 seconds or until smooth.
3. Pour into tall glasses and serve.

# Vietnamese Coffee Protein Shake

Serves: 2

## Nutritional values per serving:

- Calories – 290
- Fat – 5 g
- Carbohydrate – 31 g
- Protein – 26 g

## Ingredients:

- 1 cup almond milk, unsweetened
- 4 scoops chocolate protein power
- 4 teaspoons low fat sweetened condensed milk
- 1 cup cold chicory coffee concentrate
- 1 banana peeled, sliced, frozen

## Method:

1. Add all the ingredients into a blender.
2. Blend for 30-40 seconds or until smooth.
3. Pour into tall glasses and serve with crushed ice.

*Bring On Fitness*

# Coffee Lovers Protein Shake

Serves: 2

## Nutritional values per serving:

- Calories – 193
- Fat – 2 g
- Carbohydrate – 19 g
- Protein – 25 g

## Ingredients:

- 1 ripe banana, peeled, sliced
- 1 cup almond milk, unsweetened
- 3 cups ice cubes
- Stevia drops to taste (optional)
- 2 scoops vanilla protein powder, unsweetened
- 1 cup cold brewed coffee
- Cacao nibs to top (optional)

## Method:

1. Add banana, almond milk, ice, Stevia, protein powder and cold coffee.
2. Blend for 30-40 seconds or until smooth.
3. Pour into tall glasses and serve.

# Mocha Protein Shake

Serves: 2

## Nutritional values per serving:

- Calories – 160
- Fat – 1.5 g
- Carbohydrate – 10.8 g
- Protein – 24 g

## Ingredients:

- 1 cup nonfat milk
- 4 scoops chocolate protein powder
- 2 cups ice
- Chocolate shavings, to garnish
- 2 tablespoons Jell-O sugar free Butterscotch Pudding
- 1 cup concentrated, cold brew coffee

## Method:

1. Add milk and pudding powder into a blender and blend until well combined. It would have thickened.
2. Add protein powder, coffee and ice.
3. Blend for 30-40 seconds or until smooth. Pour into glasses.
4. Sprinkle chocolate shavings on top and serve.

*Bring On Fitness*

# Chocolate Raspberry Chia Shake

Serves: 2

## Nutritional values per serving:

- Calories – 300
- Fat – 10 g
- Carbohydrate – 33 g
- Protein – 33 g

## Ingredients:

- 2 cups water
- 1 cup frozen raspberries
- 2 tablespoons cocoa powder, unsweetened
- Cacao nibs to garnish
- Hemp seeds to garnish
- 4 scoops chocolate protein powder
- 2 tablespoons chia seeds
- ¼ teaspoon ground cinnamon

## Method:

1. Add all the ingredients into a blender.
2. Blend for about 30-40 seconds or until smooth.
3. Pour into tall glasses and serve with crushed ice.

# Chocolate Peanut Butter Smoothie

Serves: 2

## Nutritional values per serving:

- Calories – 347
- Fat – 17 g
- Carbohydrate – 19 g
- Protein – 33 g

## Ingredients:

- 2 tablespoons cocoa powder
- 2 scoops chocolate whey protein powder
- Water, as required
- 2 tablespoons natural peanut butter

## Method:

1. Add all the ingredients into a blender.
2. Blend for 30-40 seconds or until smooth.
3. Pour into tall glasses and serve.

*Bring On Fitness*

# Chapter Three: Breakfast Shakes

## Greek Goddess Banana Oat Protein Shake

Serves: 2

**Nutritional values per serving:**

- Calories – 255
- Fat – 3.4 g
- Carbohydrate – 23.4 g
- Protein – 19.8 g

**Ingredients:**

- 2 medium ripe bananas, peeled, sliced
- 2 tablespoons flaxseeds
- 1 cup water
- ½ cup steel cut oats
- 3 cups vanilla Greek yogurt

**Method:**

1. Add bananas, flaxseeds, water, oats and yogurt into the blender.
2. Blend for 30-40 seconds or until smooth.
3. Pour into tall glasses and serve.

## French Toast Shake

Serves: 2

**Nutritional values per serving:**

- Calories – 180
- Fat – 0 g
- Carbohydrate – 7 g
- Protein – 36 g

**Ingredients:**

- 1 cup fat free cottage cheese
- 2 teaspoons maple extract or 4 tablespoons sugar free maple syrup
- ¼ teaspoon nutmeg or pumpkin pie spice
- 1-2 cups water
- 1 teaspoon xanthan gum (optional)
- 2 scoops vanilla protein powder
- 1 teaspoon cinnamon powder
- Stevia powder to taste
- Ice cubes, as required
- 1 teaspoon butter extract (optional)

**Method:**

1. Add all the ingredients into a blender.
2. Blend for 30-40 seconds or until smooth.
3. Pour into tall glasses and serve.

# Blueberry Breakfast Shake

Serves: 2

**Nutritional values per serving:**

- Calories – 536
- Fat – 18 g
- Carbohydrate – 59 g
- Protein – 42 g

**Ingredients:**

- 2 cups blueberries
- 3 scoops protein powder
- ¼ cup oats
- 1 banana, peeled, sliced
- 4 tablespoons walnuts
- 2 tablespoons chia seeds

**Method:**

1. Add blueberries, protein powder, oats, banana, walnuts and chia seeds into a blender.
2. Blend for 30-40 seconds or until smooth.
3. Pour into tall glasses and serve with crushed ice.

## Chocolate Peanut Butter Banana Breakfast Shake

Serves: 2

**Nutritional values per serving:**

- Calories – 376
- Fat – 19.2 g
- Carbohydrate – 27.7 g
- Protein – 11.1 g

**Ingredients:**

- 4 large very ripe bananas, peeled, sliced, frozen
- 1 ½ cups ice
- 4 tablespoons cocoa powder, unsweetened
- 2 cups almond milk
- ½ cup creamy peanut butter
- 1 teaspoon vanilla extract

**Method:**

1. Add bananas, ice, cocoa, milk, peanut butter and vanilla extract into a blender.
2. Blend for 30-40 seconds or until smooth.
3. Pour into tall glasses and serve.

## Apple and Great Gains Shake

Serves: 2

**Nutritional values per serving:**

- Calories – 535
- Fat – 13 g
- Carbohydrate – 46 g
- Protein – 58 g

**Ingredients:**

- 1 ½ cups water
- 2 apples, cored, sliced
- 4 tablespoons almonds
- Ice cubes, as required
- 4 scoops vanilla protein powder
- 2 cups spinach
- ½ cup uncooked oats
- ½ teaspoon ground cinnamon

**Method:**

1. Add water, apples, almonds, ice, protein powder, spinach, oats and cinnamon into a blender.
2. Blend for 30-40 seconds or until smooth.
3. Pour into tall glasses and serve.

*Bring On Fitness*

# Chia Seed Piña Colada

Serves: 2

## Nutritional values per serving:

- Calories – 289
- Fat – 15 g
- Carbohydrate – 24 g
- Protein – 16 g

## Ingredients:

- 2 tablespoons chia seeds
- 2 cups frozen pineapple chunks
- 2 teaspoons flaked coconut
- 2 lime wedges, to garnish (optional)
- 2 cups coconut milk
- 1 cup Greek yogurt
- 2 teaspoons coconut oil (optional)

## Method:

1. Add all the ingredients into a blender.
2. Blend for 30-40 seconds or until smooth.
3. Pour into tall glasses and serve.

# Chapter Four: Dessert Shakes

## Key Lime Pie Protein Shake

Serves: 2

**Nutritional values per serving:**

- Calories – 180
- Fat – 0 g
- Carbohydrate – 7 g
- Protein – 36 g

**Ingredients:**

- 1 cup fat free cottage cheese
- 2 tablespoons sugar free vanilla instant pudding mix
- 1-2 cups water
- 1 teaspoon xanthan gum (optional)
- 2 scoops vanilla whey protein powder
- 2 tablespoons lime juice
- 4-6 drops green food coloring or a large handful spinach
- Stevia powder to taste
- Ice cubes, as required
- 2 graham crackers, crushed

*Bring On Fitness*

## Method:

1. Add cottage cheese, pudding mix, water, xanthan gum, protein powder, lime juice, food coloring, Stevia and ice into a blender.
2. Blend for 30-40 seconds or until smooth.
3. Pour into tall glasses and serve garnished with graham crackers.

## Vanilla Pumpkin Pie Shake

Serves: 2

**Nutritional values per serving:**

- Calories – 535
- Fat – 13 g
- Carbohydrate – 45 g
- Protein – 60 g

**Ingredients:**

- 1 ½ cups water
- 1 ½ cups pureed pumpkin
- 2 tablespoons ground flaxseeds
- 4 scoops vanilla whey protein powder
- 2 tablespoons walnuts
- 1 cup uncooked oats

**Method:**

1. Add water, pumpkin puree, flaxseeds, protein powder, walnuts and oats into a blender.
2. Blend for 30-40 seconds or until smooth.
3. Pour into tall glasses.
4. Chill for a while and serve.

## Black Forest Protein Shake

Serves: 2

### Nutritional values per serving:

- Calories – 379
- Fat – 3.9 g
- Carbohydrate – 53 g
- Protein – 37.2 g

### Ingredients:

- 4 scoops chocolate whey protein powder
- 2 bananas, peeled, sliced
- Ice cubes, as required
- 2 cups almond milk or soy milk or skim milk
- 2 heaping cups frozen dark sweet cherries, pitted

### Method:

1. Add all the ingredients into a blender.
2. Blend for 30-40 seconds or until smooth.
3. Pour into tall glasses and serve.

# High Protein Oreo Milkshake

Serves: 4

**Nutritional values per serving:**

- Calories – 211
- Fat – 3.3 g
- Carbohydrate – 24 g
- Protein – 19 g

**Ingredients:**

- 1.1 pounds fat free cottage cheese, low sodium
- 6 Oreo cookies
- 2 teaspoons vanilla extract
- 2 cups skim milk
- 2 teaspoons Truvia

**Method:**

1. Add cottage cheese, milk, cookies, Truvia and vanilla extract into a blender.
2. Blend for 30-40 seconds or until smooth.
3. Pour into tall glasses and chill for an hour.
4. Serve.

*Bring On Fitness*

# Orange Julius

Serves: 4

**Nutritional values per serving:**

- Calories – 130
- Fat – 2 g
- Carbohydrate – 15 g
- Protein – 16 g

**Ingredients:**

- 2 cups low fat cottage cheese
- Juice of 2 oranges, approximately ½ cup
- Zest of 2 oranges, grated
- 2 cups frozen strawberries
- Stevia powder to taste
- 1-2 cups ice
- 1 teaspoon vanilla extract
- 2 cups almond milk, unsweetened

**Method:**

1. Add cottage cheese, milk, orange, zest, strawberries, Stevia, ice and vanilla extract into a blender.
2. Blend for 30-40 seconds or until smooth.
3. Pour into tall glasses and serve.

# Oatmeal Raisin "Cookie" in a Glass

Serves: 2

**Nutritional values per serving:**

- Calories – 300
- Fat – 6 g
- Carbohydrate – 34 g
- Protein – 27 g

**Ingredients:**

- 2 cups almond milk, unsweetened
- 1 banana, peeled, sliced, frozen
- 2 tablespoons raisins
- ¼ teaspoon ground nutmeg
- 4 scoops vanilla protein powder
- 4 tablespoons quick cooking rolled oats
- ½ teaspoon ground cinnamon
- A pinch sea salt

**Method:**

1. Add all the ingredients into a blender.
2. Blend for 30-40 seconds or until smooth.
3. Pour into tall glasses and serve.

## Orange Creamsicle

Serves: 2

### Nutritional values per serving:

- Calories – 399
- Fat – 14 g
- Carbohydrate – 39 g
- Protein – 32 g

### Ingredients:

- 2 scoops vanilla protein powder
- ½ orange peel, grated
- 2 oranges, peeled, separated into segments, deseeded
- 2 tablespoons walnuts
- 2 cups water
- Ice cubes, as required
- 4 tablespoon flaxseed meal
- 1 cup orange juice

### Method:

1. Add all the ingredients into a blender.
2. Blend for 30-40 seconds or until smooth.
3. Pour into tall glasses and serve.

# Chapter Five: Nut Based Shakes

## Peanut Butter – Banana Shake

Serves: 2

### Nutritional values per serving:

- Calories – 366
- Fat – 16.5 g
- Carbohydrate – 40 g
- Protein – 18 g

### Ingredients:

- 1 cup fat free plain yogurt
- 1 cup fat free milk
- ½ ripe banana, preferably over ripe banana, peeled, chopped
- ¼ cup creamy peanut butter, unsalted
- 2 tablespoons honey
- Ice cubes, as required

### Method:

1. Add milk, yogurt, banana, peanut butter, honey and ice into a blender.
2. Blend for 30-40 seconds or until smooth.
3. Pour into a tall glass and serve.

## Very Berry Super Shake

Serves: 2

**Nutritional values per serving:**

- Calories – 500
- Fat – 11 g
- Carbohydrate – 54 g
- Protein – 57 g

**Ingredients:**

- 3 cups water
- 4 cups frozen mixed berries
- 2 cups spinach
- 1 cup low fat plain yogurt
- 2 tablespoons ground flaxseeds
- 2 tablespoons walnuts
- 4 scoops vanilla protein powder

**Method:**

1. Add water, berries, spinach, yogurt, flaxseeds, walnuts and protein powder into a blender and blend for 30-40 seconds or until smooth.
2. Pour into tall glasses and serve with crushed ice.

*Protein Shakes*

# Peachy Keen Smoothie

Serves: 2

## Nutritional values per serving:

- Calories – 194
- Fat – 4 g
- Carbohydrate – 17.7 g
- Protein – 17.7 g

## Ingredients:

- 4 medium ripe peaches
- 12 almonds, chopped
- 2 cups soy milk
- 2 tablespoons flax seeds
- 3 cups vanilla flavored Greek yogurt

## Method:

1. Add peaches, almonds, milk, flaxseeds and yogurt into a blender.
2. Blend for 30-40 seconds or until smooth.
3. Pour into tall glasses. Serve with crushed ice.

*Bring On Fitness*

# Peanut Butter and Jelly Protein Smoothie

Serves: 2

## Nutritional values per serving:

- Calories – 417
- Fat – 11 g
- Carbohydrate – 41 g
- Protein – 41 g

## Ingredients:

- 2 cups mixed frozen berries
- ½ cup vanilla whey protein powder
- 2 cups milk of your choice
- 2-4 tablespoons natural peanut butter
- 4 tablespoons rolled oats

## Method:

1. Add milk, peanut butter, protein powder, oats and berries into a blender.
2. Blend for 30-40 seconds or until smooth.
3. Pour into tall glasses.
4. Chill for an hour and serve.

# Chocolate, Peanut Butter and Banana

Serves: 2

## Nutritional values per serving: With water

- Calories – 585
- Fat – 22 g
- Carbohydrate – 38 g
- Protein – 59 g

## Ingredients:

- 3 cups water or milk or yogurt
- 2 bananas, peeled, sliced
- 4 tablespoons natural peanut butter
- 4 scoops chocolate protein powder
- 2 cups spinach, torn
- 2 tablespoons cacao nibs or dark cocoa powder

## Method:

1. Add water / milk, peanut butter, protein powder, bananas, spinach and cacao nibs into a blender.
2. Blend for 30-40 seconds or until smooth.
3. Pour into tall glasses.
4. Chill for an hour and serve.

## Apple Shake

Serves: 2

**Nutritional values per serving:**

- Calories – 482
- Fat – 16.5 g
- Carbohydrate – 71 g
- Protein – 19 g

**Ingredients:**

- 2 medium apples, peeled, chopped
- 1 cup skim milk or soy milk
- 2 teaspoons apple pie spice
- 4 tablespoons cashew butter
- 12 ounce vanilla yogurt
- Ice cubes, as required

**Method:**

1. Add apples, milk, spice, cashew butter, yogurt and ice into a blender.
2. Blend for 30-40 seconds or until smooth.
3. Pour into tall glasses and serve.

# Coconut and Almond Shake

Serves: 4

## Nutritional values per serving:

- Calories – 405
- Fat – 21 g
- Carbohydrate – 33 g
- Protein – 27 g

## Ingredients:

- 3 tablespoons almond butter
- 2 scoops chocolate protein powder
- 2 cups dark chocolate almond milk
- 3 cups water
- 2 tablespoons coconut flakes, unsweetened
- Ice cubes, as required

## Method:

1. Add all the ingredients into a blender.
2. Blend for 30-40 seconds or until smooth.
3. Pour into tall glasses and serve.

*Bring On Fitness*

# Almond Butter Chia Shake

Serves: 2

## Nutritional values per serving:

- Calories – 280
- Fat – 14 g
- Carbohydrate – 39 g
- Protein – 7.5 g

## Ingredients:

- 2 large ripe bananas, frozen
- 2 tablespoons almond butter
- 1 ½ cups almond milk
- 2 tablespoons chia seeds

## Method:

1. Add all the ingredients into a blender.
2. Blend for 30-40 seconds or until smooth.
3. Pour into tall glasses and serve.

# Chapter Six: Vegan Shakes

## Peanut Butter Cup

Serves: 2

### Nutritional values per serving:

- Calories – 258
- Fat – 6 g
- Carbohydrate – 21 g
- Protein – 30 g

### Ingredients:

- 1 cup almond milk, unsweetened
- 2 tablespoons cocoa powder, unsweetened
- 1 tablespoon natural peanut butter, unsalted
- 2 scoops plant based vanilla or chocolate protein powder
- 1 banana, peeled, sliced, frozen
- Water, as required

### Method:

1. Add water, milk, peanut butter, protein powder, bananas and cocoa powder into a blender.
2. Blend for 30-40 seconds or until smooth.
3. Pour into tall glasses and serve.

*Bring On Fitness*

# Vanilla Chai

Serves: 2

### Nutritional values per serving:

- Calories – 219
- Fat – 9 g
- Carbohydrate – 20 g
- Protein – 17 g

### Ingredients:

- ½ cup almond milk, unsweetened
- 1 teaspoon ground cinnamon
- ½ cup chai tea (brewed using 2 tea bags, chilled)
- 1 tablespoon natural almond butter, unsalted
- 1 scoops plant based vanilla protein powder
- 1 banana, peeled, sliced, frozen
- Water, as required

### Method:

1. Add water, milk, chai tea, almond butter, protein powder, bananas and cinnamon into a blender.
2. Blend for 30-40 seconds or until smooth.
3. Pour into tall glasses and serve.

# Dark Chocolate Peppermint Protein Shake

Serves: 2

**Nutritional values per serving:**

- Calories – 296
- Fat – 6 g
- Carbohydrate – 49 g
- Protein – 22 g

**Ingredients:**

- 2 large bananas, peeled, sliced, frozen
- 2 cups non-dairy milk of your choice
- 4 tablespoons cacao powder
- 2 tablespoons dark vegan chocolate chips
- 2 scoops plant based chocolate protein powder
- ½ teaspoon pure peppermint extract
- Ice cubes, as required
- 1/8 teaspoon sea salt

For topping:

- Vegan whipped topping

**Method:**

1. Add all the ingredients into a blender.
2. Blend for 30-40 seconds or until smooth.
3. Pour into tall glasses and serve topped with whipped topping.

## Green Monster

Serves: 2

**Nutritional values per serving:**

- Calories – 271
- Fat – 6 g
- Carbohydrate – 6 g
- Protein – 15 g

**Ingredients:**

- ½ cup apple juice, unsweetened
- 1 scoop plant based vanilla protein powder
- 1 cup baby spinach, loosely packed
- ½ ripe avocado, peeled, pitted, chopped
- ½ cup water
- 1 Bosc pear, cored, chopped
- 1 banana, peeled, sliced, frozen

**Method:**

1. Add all the ingredients into a blender.
2. Blend for 30-40 seconds or until smooth.
3. Pour into tall glasses and serve.

# Matcha Pear Green Protein Shake

Serves: 2

**Nutritional values per serving:**

- Calories – 289
- Fat – 9.8 g
- Carbohydrate – 34.3 g
- Protein – 22.5 g

**Ingredients:**

- 2 scoops plant based vanilla protein powder
- 2 cups spinach
- 1 teaspoon matcha tea powder
- 2 cups almond milk, unsweetened
- 2 pears, cored, sliced

**Method:**

1. Add all the ingredients into a blender.
2. Blend for 30-40 seconds or until smooth.
3. Pour into tall glasses and serve.

*Bring On Fitness*

# Baked Apple Shake

Serves: 2

### Nutritional values per serving: With water

- Calories – 510
- Fat – 15 g
- Carbohydrate – 36 g
- Protein – 57 g

### Ingredients:

- 2 apples, cored, sliced into wedges
- 3 cups water or dairy free milk
- 2 cups spinach, torn
- 2 tablespoons ground flaxseeds
- ½ teaspoon ground cinnamon
- 4 scoops plant based vanilla protein powder
- 2 tablespoons almonds, chopped
- 2 tablespoons sesame seeds

### Method:

1. Add all the ingredients into a blender.
2. Blend for 30-40 seconds or until smooth.
3. Pour into tall glasses and serve.

# Toasted Coconut Protein Shake

Serves: 2

**Nutritional values per serving:**

- Calories – 305
- Fat – 18 g
- Carbohydrate – 14 g
- Protein – 25 g

**Ingredients:**

- 2 cups coconut milk, unsweetened
- ½ cup coconut flakes, unsweetened, toasted until golden brown.
- 4 scoops plant based vanilla protein powder
- 2 cups ice

**Method:**

1. Add all the ingredients into a blender.
2. Blend for 30-40 seconds or until smooth.
3. Pour into tall glasses and serve.

*Bring On Fitness*

# Conclusion

With that, we have come to the end of this book. The recipes in this book will set you on the right path to achieving the body that you have always dreamed of and help you lose weight in a healthy manner.

All the recipes are tried, tested and tasted; and are delicious, refreshing and nutritious, as well as being diet-friendly. You will be able to drink them without feeling guilty and all of these can be used as meal replacements.

The recipes are quite versatile and can be modified as per your requirements. For instance, if you want to replace certain ingredients or remove items, you can do it. Before replacing an ingredient or adding a new one, it is recommended to check whether the ingredient aligns with your current diet or not.

Thank you, and remember to share how well these weight loss protein shake recipes work for you. You can do that by writing a review in your Amazon account under Your Orders.

Thank you,

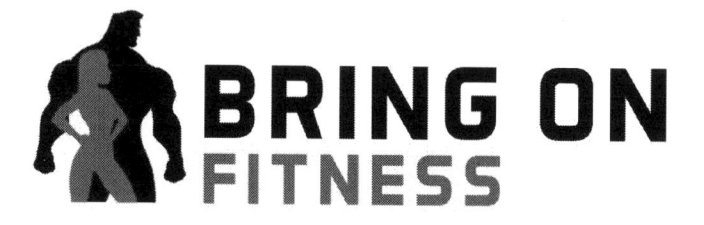

**BRING ON FITNESS**

Printed in Great Britain
by Amazon